# YOUR KNOWLEDGE HAS VALUE

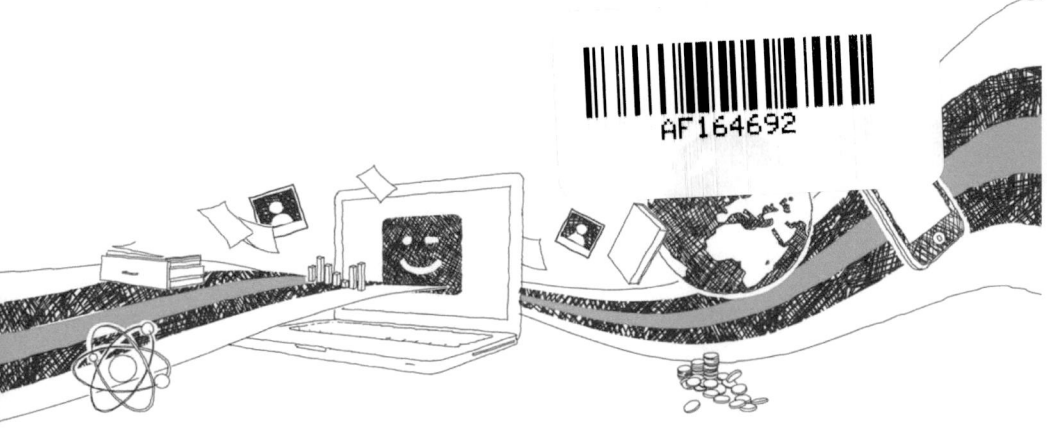

- We will publish your bachelor's and master's thesis, essays and papers

- Your own eBook and book - sold worldwide in all relevant shops

- Earn money with each sale

Upload your text at www.GRIN.com and publish for free

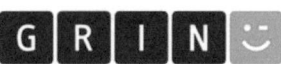

**Bibliographic information published by the German National Library:**

The German National Library lists this publication in the National Bibliography; detailed bibliographic data are available on the Internet at http://dnb.dnb.de .

This book is copyright material and must not be copied, reproduced, transferred, distributed, leased, licensed or publicly performed or used in any way except as specifically permitted in writing by the publishers, as allowed under the terms and conditions under which it was purchased or as strictly permitted by applicable copyright law. Any unauthorized distribution or use of this text may be a direct infringement of the author s and publisher s rights and those responsible may be liable in law accordingly.

**Imprint:**

Copyright © 2018 GRIN Verlag
Print and binding: Books on Demand GmbH, Norderstedt Germany
ISBN: 9783668627628

**This book at GRIN:**

https://www.grin.com/document/388764

Patrick Kimuyu

# The Role of Managed Care Organizations within the Healthcare Industry

GRIN Verlag

**GRIN - Your knowledge has value**

Since its foundation in 1998, GRIN has specialized in publishing academic texts by students, college teachers and other academics as e-book and printed book. The website www.grin.com is an ideal platform for presenting term papers, final papers, scientific essays, dissertations and specialist books.

**Visit us on the internet:**

http://www.grin.com/

http://www.facebook.com/grincom

http://www.twitter.com/grin_com

## Contents

Introduction .................................................................................................................................... 2
Overview of Managed Care Organizations .................................................................................... 2
    Managed Care Principles .......................................................................................................... 3
Managed Care Compared to Conventional Health Care ............................................................... 4
Types of Managed Care and what They Are .................................................................................. 5
    Health Maintenance Organizations (HMO) .............................................................................. 5
    Preferred Provider Organizations (PPOs) ................................................................................. 6
    Point-of-Service (POS) Plans ..................................................................................................... 7
Advantages of Managed Care ........................................................................................................ 7
    Decreased Cost ......................................................................................................................... 8
    Accredited Care ........................................................................................................................ 8
    Large In-Network Providers ..................................................................................................... 9
    Cheaper Prescriptions .............................................................................................................. 9
Disadvantages of Managed Care ................................................................................................... 9
    Restricted Care ......................................................................................................................... 9
    Out-Of-Network Providers ..................................................................................................... 10
    Lack of Specialty Care ............................................................................................................ 10
    Increased Cost of Unapproved Care ...................................................................................... 10
    No Access for the Uninsured .................................................................................................. 11
    Strict Approval Processes ....................................................................................................... 11
    Referral Issues ........................................................................................................................ 11
Summary ...................................................................................................................................... 11
References ................................................................................................................................... 13

## Introduction

Over the decades, the United States' healthcare system has been experiencing challenges. In general, the cost and quality of care has always been considered as the most critical factors that influence healthcare sustainability in the United States and the world, as a whole. As a result, a series of value-based payment reforms have been introduced. For instance, the Affordable Care Act (ACA) of 2010 introduced payment and delivery system reforms. From a critical perspective, the reforms introduced by the ACA have addressed the long-standing problems which have been posing enormous hindrances to the development of the U.S. healthcare system (Lewis, Colla, Carluzzo, Kler & Fisher, 2013). Above all, it has enhanced managed care through consolidating care, as well as, addressing the problem of unsustainable costs and uneven quality of care. However, managed care seems to exhibit some drawbacks too. Therefore, this paper will provide a comprehensive overview of managed care, primarily on the advantages and disadvantages of managed care organizations.

## Overview of Managed Care Organizations

Managed care seems to have gained widespread acceptance by states over the past two decades. This phenomenon is attributable to several reasons. Foremost, the integration of managed care into Medicaid programs has enabled states to control costs associated with the program (O'Connell, 2011). It is also apparent that managed care has enhanced service utilization within the U.S. healthcare system. This implies that managed care organizations have been instrumental in the implementation of value-based payment reforms.

Historically, managed care organizations have existed for almost half decade. The emergence of managed care organizations dates back to 1973 when the Health Maintenance Organization Act was passed by the Congress. Consequently, the Health Maintenance

Organizations (HMOs) emerged as the first for model of managed care. This was followed by the formation of other managed care organizations. These managed care organizations exhibited distinctions in various aspects. Wagner & Kongstvedt (2007) reaffirm that reasonable distinctions between various types of managed care organizations were explicit. However, this aspect has changed significantly to a point where it is difficult to differentiate between managed care organizations and insurance companies. Despite the existence of managed care organizations two decades ago or longer, the conventional healthcare model or the fee-for-service model dominated healthcare delivery in the U.S. care system. Instead, managed care organizations were considered as 'alternative delivery systems.' However, there has been a significant paradigm shift over the past two decades that has seen managed care organizations become the dominant form of health insurance coverage across the nation. It is reported that only few people remain covered under the traditional fee-for-service model (Wagner & Kongstvedt, 2007).

## Managed Care Principles

In retrospect, it is apparent that managed care has evolved over years into its current form. This evolution seems to have been occurred due to forces in the purchaser delivery system. As a result, virtually all managed care organizations appear relatively the same without, especially on the basis of operational principles. In the current situation, managed care organizations manage care of Medicaid enrollees through the U.S. healthcare system that plays various responsibilities.

Foremost, the managed care system is responsible for coordinating and monitoring primary care, primarily through tertiary services. Second, the managed care system facilitates prevention and health education. Third, it ensures that the concerned population receives care in appropriate setting. As such, it is responsible for ensuring that enrollees to these programs receive care from appropriate healthcare providers. For instance, specialists versus primary care specialists or hospitals versus outpatient clinics. Finally, the system is responsible for aligning incentives, in order to promote cost-effectiveness in care provision. Some of the key approaches for achieving cost-effectiveness include cost-sharing and capitation of providers (Sekhri, 2000).

## Managed Care Compared to Conventional Health Care

It is apparent that managed care and the conventional healthcare models exhibit differences. Some of the key differences include the quality of care, payment for care and the way enrollees choose physicians. Overall, managed care organizations adopt the managed care model which is reasonably distinct from the traditional fee-for-service model. One of the most outstanding characteristics of managed care organizations is the limitation of access to services by enrollees. In this context, they operate under a comprehensive systems; 'capitated' systems. 'Capitated' systems involve the contraction of a private company to oversee enrollees' healthcare services. In this case, the private company assumes the financial risk associated with health insurance coverage. Under this system, a managed care organization is responsible for establishing its network of healthcare providers who provide services to Medicaid enrollees. Consequently, the state sets the total amount of money for enrollees that it pays the managed care organization. In this case, the organization bears all the financial risk related to coverage. However, its provision of care to Medicaid enrollees is limited within the state's fixed cost (O'Connell, 2011).

On the other hand, the conventional healthcare model or the 'primary care case management' system involves the coordination of enrollees' care by a paid healthcare provider, but financial risk of coverage is retained by the state. Under this system, the state reimburses

Medicaid providers, primarily on the basis of fee-for-service precepts. As such, enrollees in this program can only receive care from a specified primary care provider. Overall, both systems focus on controlling the cost of care for Medicaid enrollees (O'Connell, 2011).

Regarding the quality of care, the managed care model provides the best care compared to the conventional healthcare model. The fact that enrollees are free to choose their preferred healthcare provider within the network implies that only receive satisfactory care from the best providers. In another perspective, the collective provision of care to a specified population group attracts competition among healthcare providers, an aspect that has always been associated with improved quality of care.

## Types of Managed Care and what They Are

In general, there are different forms of managed care organizations. These programs are network-based, meaning that care is provided to Medicaid enrollees within a specified scope of providers' network. Therefore, they exhibit differences in the levels of restriction with some of the programs being highly restrictive whereas others are less restrictive with regard to the specific network. Currently, there are three main types of managed care organizations: Health Maintenance Organizations (HMO), Preferred Provider Organizations (PPO) and Point-of-Service (POS) plans.

### Health Maintenance Organizations (HMO)

Health Maintenance Organizations refers to organized healthcare systems. These healthcare systems provide a wide range of health services to the specific population that is enrolled into Medicaid programs. In addition, they provide financing for care provision to enrollees. As such, an HMO acts as a combination of management system responsible healthcare delivery and a health insurer. In principle, these organizations coordinate or provide healthcare services to enrollees in the program, primarily through affiliated healthcare providers. These healthcare providers are then reimbursed through various platforms, unlike in the traditional health insurance coverage plan where insurance companies reimburse enrollees for their healthcare cost. On the other hand, HMOs ensure appropriateness and quality of health services that they offer to members within their networks (Sekhri, 2000).

However, it is worth noting that HMOs adopt different models. The most common HMO models include group model, network model, direct contract model, staff model, and independent practice association (IPA) model. In the U.S., group and network HMO models are the most popular. Group model HMOs involves the provision of healthcare services to enrollees though a multispecialty physician group that is contracted by HMO. These physicians are required to treat HMO members, although the model allows them to attend to other patients outside the HMO system. Outstanding examples of HMO group models are the Kaiser Foundation Health Plan that contracts the Permanente Medical Groups, particularly in California, and the Geisinger Health Plan of Danville that has contractual relationship with Geisinger Clinic, in Pennsylvania (Sekhri, 2000).

On the other hand, a network model involves the provision of health services to members of HMO program by more than one group practice contracted by HMO. Health Insurance Plan (HIP) of Greater New York serves as an outstanding example of this kind of HMO. HIP has established contractual relationship with numerous physician group practices in New York (Sekhri, 2000).

## Preferred Provider Organizations (PPOs)

Preferred provider organizations refer to care entities through which enrollees in a selected network are given healthcare services that are purchased through a contract between a

# BEI GRIN MACHT SICH IHR WISSEN BEZAHLT

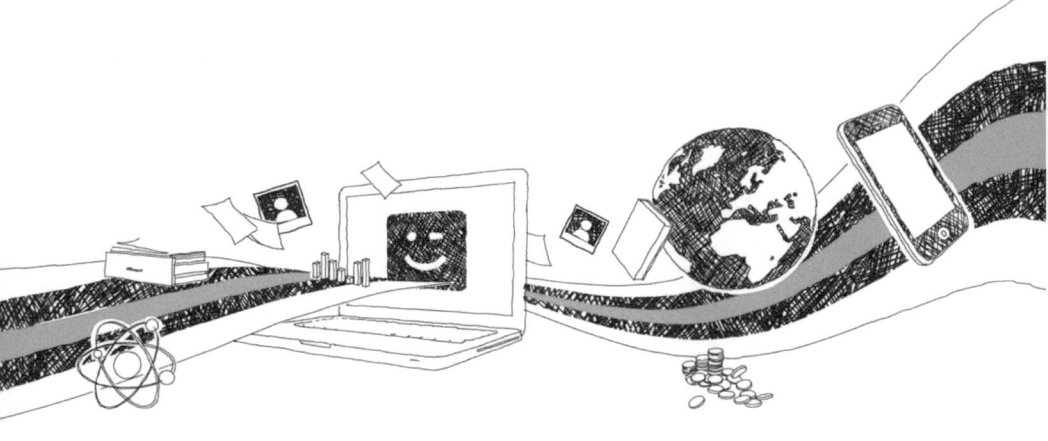

- Wir veröffentlichen Ihre Hausarbeit, Bachelor- und Masterarbeit

- Ihr eigenes eBook und Buch - weltweit in allen wichtigen Shops

- Verdienen Sie an jedem Verkauf

Jetzt bei www.GRIN.com hochladen und kostenlos publizieren

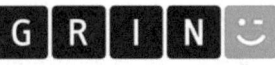

**Bibliografische Information der Deutschen Nationalbibliothek:**

Die Deutsche Bibliothek verzeichnet diese Publikation in der Deutschen Nationalbibliografie; detaillierte bibliografische Daten sind im Internet über http://dnb.d-nb.de/ abrufbar.

Dieses Werk sowie alle darin enthaltenen einzelnen Beiträge und Abbildungen sind urheberrechtlich geschützt. Jede Verwertung, die nicht ausdrücklich vom Urheberrechtsschutz zugelassen ist, bedarf der vorherigen Zustimmung des Verlages. Das gilt insbesondere für Vervielfältigungen, Bearbeitungen, Übersetzungen, Mikroverfilmungen, Auswertungen durch Datenbanken und für die Einspeicherung und Verarbeitung in elektronische Systeme. Alle Rechte, auch die des auszugsweisen Nachdrucks, der fotomechanischen Wiedergabe (einschließlich Mikrokopie) sowie der Auswertung durch Datenbanken oder ähnliche Einrichtungen, vorbehalten.

**Impressum:**

Copyright © 2017 GRIN Verlag
Druck und Bindung: Books on Demand GmbH, Norderstedt Germany
ISBN: 9783668625099

**Dieses Buch bei GRIN:**

https://www.grin.com/document/385950

12. WHO handbook on indoor radon: a public health perspective/ edited by Hajo Zeeb and Ferid Shannon 2009
13. Sources and effects of ionizing radiation: UNSCEAR 1995 report to the General Assembly, with Scientific Annexes. United Nations New York, 1994 (p. 80)
14. Darby S, et al. Radon in homes and risk of lung cancer: collaborative analysis of individual date from 13 European case-control studies. Br. Med. J. 330: 223-227, 2005
15. Stix C. et al. Case-control study on childhood cancer in the vicinity of nuclear power plants in Germany 1980-2003. European Journal of Cancer 44: 275-284, 2008
16. Cardis E. et al. "Estimates of the Cancer Burden in Europe from Radioactive Fallout from Chernobyl Accident." International Journal of Cancer, 199:1224-1235, 2006
17. Bardi J. "Chernobyl Cleanup Workers Had Significantly Increased Risk of Leukemia". Univ. of California at San Francisco News, November 8, 2012.
18. Bolonov M. The Chernobyl accident as a source of new radiological knowledge: implications for Fukushima rehabilitation and research programmes. J. Radiol.Prot.33: 27-40, 2013

mailto: hans.grasmuk@A1.net

# BEI GRIN MACHT SICH IHR WISSEN BEZAHLT

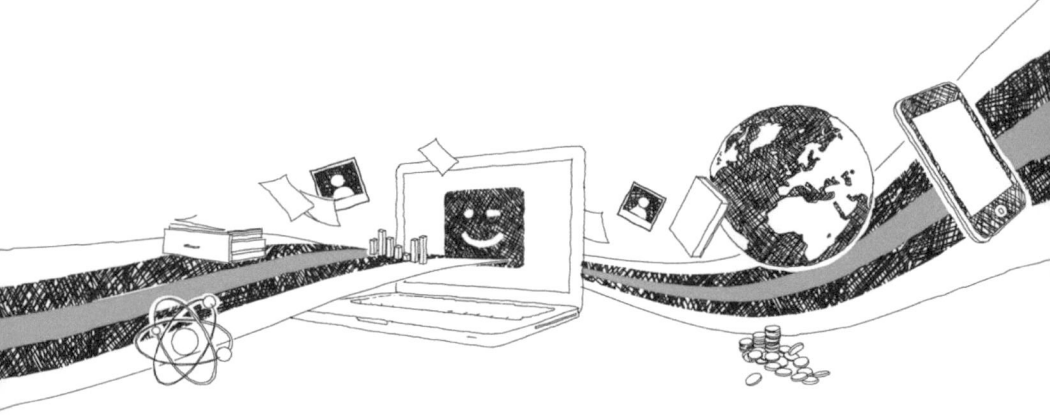

- Wir veröffentlichen Ihre Hausarbeit, Bachelor- und Masterarbeit

- Ihr eigenes eBook und Buch - weltweit in allen wichtigen Shops

- Verdienen Sie an jedem Verkauf

Jetzt bei www.GRIN.com hochladen und kostenlos publizieren

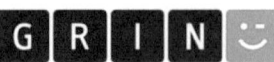

health insurance carrier and employer health benefit plan. In this network, the PPO develops payment levels and reimbursement procedures that are accepted by the participating healthcare providers. Unlike HMOs, PPOs allow their members to use non-PPO providers. However, this attracts higher levels of deductibles for members. Despite the differences observed in PPOs, especially those who operate on specialty-only basis, they all share common characteristics regarding provider network, utilization management, consumer choice, and negotiated payment rates. In most cases, PPOs establish contractual relationships with physicians and hospitals, either directly or indirectly based on providers' scope of services, community reputation and cost-effectiveness. On the other hand, PPOs control the cost and utilization of health services through implementing appropriate utilization management strategies. Moreover, PPOs involve full payment for health services covered at negotiated payment rates. As such, participating providers must agree to PPOs payment rates (Sekhri, 2000).

## Point-of-Service (POS) Plans

In practice, POS utilizes other programs, especially HMO-like health plans. It combines indemnity coverage with these health plans, especially in covering health services that are offered to members of the particular plans outside their networks. One of the main features of POS is that the plan does not allow members to choose their preferred system until the point of service use. This type of MCOs is gaining popularity due to their flexibility.

## Advantages of Managed Care

In retrospect, managed care has been found to generate several benefits. Some of the most common benefits of managed care system include low cost, provision of accredited care, cheaper prescriptions, and the availability of extensive in-network providers.

## Decreased Cost

Ideally, managed care programs are adopted as value-based payment reforms that are aimed at reducing the cost of healthcare. At the national scope, the cost of healthcare in the U.S. can be analyzed from the perspective of the country's report on national health expenditures. In retrospect, it is apparent that the adoption of a managed care system has led to an historical cost reduction in 51-year history. According to Centers for Medicare and Medicaid Services [CMS] (2013), there has been a significant decrease in healthcare costs in the past decade. For instance, 2011 recorded a remarkable decrease of Medicaid spending per beneficiary which was estimated at 0.9%. Concisely, the trend of increasing family premiums has reversed. Reports indicate that the annual family premiums had reached 6.2% by 2008, but it decreased to 4.5% in 2012 (CMS, 2013). This significant decrease in family premiums for insured populations indicates that managed care has led to decreased cost in the system.

## Accredited Care

Accredited care is the second advantage of managed care. Foremost, it is worth noting that managed care organizations establish accreditation procedures that must be met by all the providers participating in the network. This ensures that all providers are providing high quality health services to members of the respective MCOs. Second, managed care is meant to be a value-based payment program. As such, high quality is emphasized over all other aspects of healthcare operations. One the key approaches that ensures accredited care is the subjection of health professionals and institutions to a rigorous accreditation process. Their experiences and credentials are analyzed carefully before approval to ascertain their innate capacity for providing quality care to members. Therefore, MCOs ensure that their beneficiaries receive healthcare services that meet high quality standards.

### Large In-Network Providers

In reality, managed care organizations involve large in-network providers. Most MCOs do not set limits for the number of healthcare providers participating in their networks. This implies that managed care provides full specialty services to enrollees of Medicaid programs. For instance, HMO provider networks are very extensive, covering a large scope of specialty practices, especially through HMO network model (Sekhri, 2000).

### Cheaper Prescriptions

Finally, managed care focuses on reducing the cost of health services for members. As such, they adopt cost-effective strategies to ensure that their members receive affordable care. Foremost, their incentives involve cheap prescriptions. Ideally, reducing the overall cost of care creates opportunities for subsidizing costs for other treatment related costs. In addition, the availability of a wide providers network within MCO's programs enable member to shop for the highest quality of care with low cost. As such, they enjoy cheaper prescriptions compared to members in the conventional healthcare system where prescriptions are expensive.

## Disadvantages of Managed Care

Despite the numerous benefits reaped from managed care, it is apparent that the system has some disadvantages. Sekhri (2000) admits that managed care has led to the emergence of several complaints. Some of the main complaints include restriction of care, lack of specialty care and increased cost of upapproved care. Other disadvantages include strict approval process, referral issues and inaccessibility to uninsured people.

### Restricted Care

Restricted care has been identified as one of the disadvantages of managed care. Ideally, states give MCOs a set total amount for the reimbursement of healthcare services offered to

Medicaid enrollees. As such, these MCOs are supposed to maintain the cost of care below the set limits. This implies that they restrict care for patients, in order to avoid going beyond the reimbursement standards (O'Connell, 2011). As a result, enrollees can only receive restricted care that corresponds to the coverage. Some MCOs exclude sicker patients, in order to avoid high cost of care (Hall, n.d.).

## Out-Of-Network Providers

Access to health services from out-of-network providers is another disadvantage associated with managed care. This system involves the provision of health services by the participating providers. Therefore, providers who are not within the network cannot offer services to MCO members. This implies that the 'capitated' system creates an unfavorable environment in the market. As a result, there are some economic consequences associated with this form of market strategy. For instance, out-of-network providers who provide health services to MCO members cannot be paid through MCO's reimbursement process.

## Lack of Specialty Care

Lack of specialty care is another significant problem of managed care. In practice, MCOs have a network of providers who, in most cases, do not provide full specialty practices. For instance, most PPOs operate on specialty-only basis. This implies that their members receive specified treatments only.

## Increased Cost of Unapproved Care

It is also apparent that managed care involves increased cost of unapproved care. In principle, members of MCOs are required to seek for health services within the specified network of providers. Therefore, members who receive health services from out-of-network providers pay increased deductibles, especially under PPO. In some circumstances, members foot their medical bills with the provider (Sekhri, 2000).

### No Access for the Uninsured

Inaccessibility to healthcare services by uninsured people through managed care is one of the greatest disadvantages. According to the managed care principles, members of MCOs are supposed to be enrolled in a health insurance plan for eligibility. Therefore, uninsured people cannot benefit from managed care (Wagner & Kongstvedt, 2007).

### Strict Approval Processes

Managed care is also associated with strict approval process. For instance, physicians participating in provider networks must meet set standards. Similarly, health facilities are scrutinized before approval to participate in MCO networks. Physicians are also supposed to comply with imposed bureaucracy and micromanaged clinical environment (Hall, n.d.).

### Referral Issues

Referral for patients is also a tricky issue under managed care. This is so because, it is difficult to refer patients to facilities outside the network due to lack of specialty care. In some circumstances, MCO members are forced to co-pay for their healthcare services obtained from non-MCO providers.

## Summary

In a brief conclusion, managed care has been found to generate enormous benefits. The main types of MCOs are MHO, PPO and POS, and they all operate under managed care principles. These forms of care system have many benefits compared to the conventional care.

Foremost, it reduces the cost of care; thus leading to a significant decrease in national health expenditure. It also facilitates provision of health services to MCO members at low premiums. On the other hand, managed care ensures provision of quality care to enrollees. Other benefits include cheaper prescriptions and the availability of extensive in-network providers.

However, managed care has some disadvantages including restriction of care, lack of specialty care and increased cost of unapproved care. Other disadvantages include strict approval process, referral issues and inaccessibility to uninsured people.

## References

CMS (2013). *Lower costs, better care: reforming our health care delivery system.* Retrieved from https://www.cms.gov/Newsroom/MediaReleaseDatabase/Fact-sheets/2013-Fact-sheets-items/2013-02-28.html

Hall, R. (n.d.). *Ethical and legal implications of managed care.* Retrieved from http://www.drrichardhall.com/Articles/ethical.pdf

Lewis, V., Colla, H., Carluzzo, K., Kler, S., & Fisher, E. (2013). Accountable care organizations in the United States: market and demographic factors associated with formation. *Health Serv Res.*, 48(6 Pt 1), 1840–1858.

http://www.ncbi.nlm.nih.gov/pmc/articles/PMC3876396/

O'Connell, S. (2011). *Medicaid monitoring an overview of managed care.* Retrieved from http://leg.mt.gov/content/Committees/Interim/2011-2012/Children-Family/Topics/Medicaid%20Monitoring/nov2011-managed-care-overview.pdf

Sekhri, N. (2000). Managed care: the US experience. *Bulletin of the World Health Organization*, 78 (6), 830-844. Retrieved from http://www.who.int/bulletin/archives/78(6)830.pdf

Wagner, E., & Kongstvedt, P. (2007). Types of managed care organizations and integrated health care delivery systems. In P. Kongstvedt (Eds.), *Essentials of managed health care* (pp. 19-40). Burlington, MA: Jones & Bartlett Learning.

# YOUR KNOWLEDGE HAS VALUE

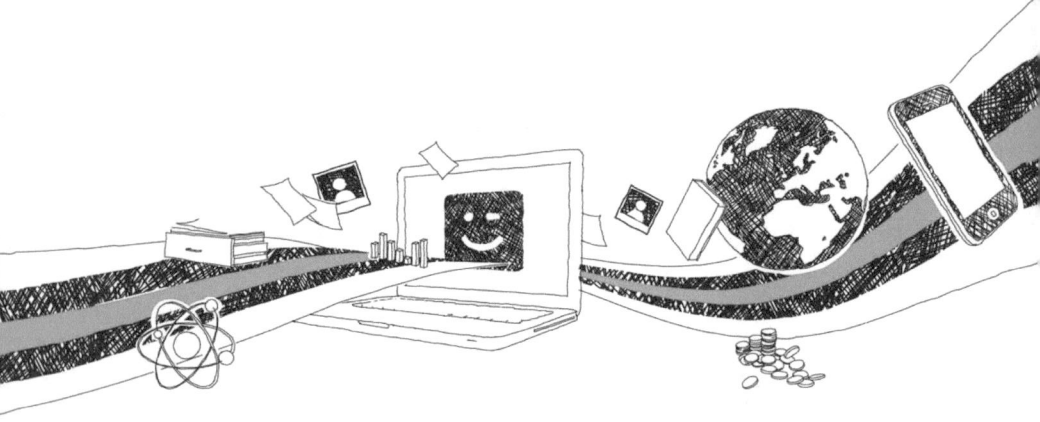

- We will publish your bachelor's and master's thesis, essays and papers

- Your own eBook and book -
  sold worldwide in all relevant shops

- Earn money with each sale

Upload your text at www.GRIN.com
and publish for free

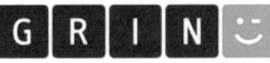